INSTANT VITAMIN-MINERAL LOCATOR

by

Hanna Kroeger

Dear Reader,

Years of acquaintance can teach us much of each other, and so it is in regard to my friend Rev. Hanna Kroeger of Boulder, Colorado.

She has proven herself to be a child of nature and has dedicated her life to its study and also its application in the field of nutrition.

This book is but a small facet of her endeavors. You who are sincerely interested in nutrition and its vital impression in the human body will find this book most rewarding.

Yours in Light and Truth,

Rev. Dr. F. Houston

CONTENTS

INTRODUCTION

A healthy body fed with healthy food is able to manufacture its own Vitamins with the exception of Vitamin C.

Healthy food is not plastic, refined, puffed up, stabilized or chemicalized for appearance, preservation or shelf life and is not over cooked or under cooked.

Healthy food is not bleached and sprayed as in cereals & grains, not green picked fruits, not meat with Diethylstilbestrol, not eggs from chickens fed with speed and hormones, not milk in cartons treated with formaldehyde.

Healthy food is just plain good food. With this plain good food the intestinal tract is able to manufacture:

> B-vitamins
> Folic acid
> Pantothenic acid
> Biotin
> Methionine
> Rutin
> Vitamin K2
> Vitamin P
> Nicotinic acid
> Converts Carotene to Vitamin A

However, the sterilization of the intestinal tract through preservatives, antibiotics and not "good" food hinders the flora from manufacturing above mentioned vitamins in sufficient amounts or in some cases completely.

Sincere efforts should be made to establish the balance of flora in the intestines by taking:

> buttermilk
> yoghurt
> sprouted foods
> acidophilus cultures
> acidophilus capsules

and by avoiding preservatives. It will take several weeks and often months to reestablish the balance.

Until the intestinal flora is functioning to full capacity all nutrients, which ordinarily are manufactured in the intestinal tract, have to be taken into the body by means of food supplements otherwise, one, two, or multiple deficiencies will arise.

How good is your flora?

PART I

Vitamins in Nutrition

Vitamin A

Vitamin A is a fat soluble vitamin which is synthesized in the human and animal body from carotene.

Carotene is called a provitamin and is changed to vitamin A in the healthy walls of the intestinal tract.

Vitamin A as such is found in meat products and lover oils such as: cod liver oil, halibut liver oil, in cream, butter and egg yolk.

The amount of Vitamin A in cream, butter and eggs varies a lot according to the seasons and feeding conditions of the animals. For example, 1/4 lb. of butter made from grazing animals has 5,000 I.U.s (international units) of Vitamin A and 16,000 I.U.s of Carotene. 1/4 lb. butter made from milk of animals fed on hay in wintertime has only 1,000 I.U.s of A and 300 I.U.s of Carotene.

Vitamin A is needed for healthy
 skin
 hair
 nails
 eyes
 lungs
 mouth and all membranes of the digestive tract
  and uro-genital organs

Vitamin A is needed for the healthy lubrication of all membranes. If membranes are dry, bacteria, virus and molds have a better chance to attack them.

Check for yourself the following symptoms and report to your physician for possible Vitamin A deficiency:
 night blindness
 impaired vision
 difficulty to adapt to darkness
 eyelids are glued in the mornings
 inability to distinguish the colors blue and yellow
 skin troubles such as:
  dryness, scaliness
  pigmentation
  dandruff

brittle hair & nails

outside of arms & legs become rough

loss of hearing

loss of taste

gastric troubles

stone formation in gallbladder and kidneys

repeated infections in nose and sinuses.

Clinically speaking

Vitamin A is used for:

1) Promoting tissue formation
2) Increasing blood platelets
3) Promoting digestion
4) Preventing senility (old age)

Folks with following conditions are unable to synthesize A from Carotene and do need an extra Vitamin A supplement:

In celiac disease

In ulcerated colitis

In obstruction of bile duct

In cirrhosis of the liver

Vitamin A cannot be stored in Hyperthyroidism and in Diabetes mellitus. Acute infections such as pneumonia, high fevers and influenza destroy Vitamin A rapidly. Unhealthy flora of the intestines also prohibits the conversion of carotene to Vitamin A.

B₁ or Thiamin

B₁ or Thiamin is No. 1 of the B Vitamin complex and can be isolated.

If following symptoms persist check with your physician and discuss with him possible thiamin deficiency.

Alcoholism
Fibrilation of eye
Edema of eye
Bleeding retina
Difficulties in rising from your knees
Delayed ligament reflexes
Listlessness
Hangover
Nausea
Constipation
Loss of muscles on lower arms and legs
Slight paralysis
Loss of stomach acidity
Lack of urination
Painful menstruation
Sciatica
Loss of morale
Loss of sense of humor
Unexplainable irritability
Nerves on edge.

B₂ or Riboflavin

B_2 (Riboflavin) is the second one of the B Vitamin complex and can be isolated. If following symptoms persist check with you physician and discuss possible Riboflavin deficiency with him.

Fissures in edge of mouth
Bright light is bothering
Eyes are reddened/are tired easily
Burning sensation under eyelids
Painful sensation under eyelids
Loss of vision at distance
Lips are painful, fissured
Muscle cramps
Red scaly spots between nose and lips
Tongue swollen/bright red/painful
Oily skin/hair
White heads
Vaginal itching
Abnormal sensation in legs
Trembling as in low blood sugar
Dizzy as in low blood sugar
Sluggish as in low blood sugar.

Riboflavin is a coferment to phosphorus and is needed for proper cell respiration

Riboflavin regulates sodium-potassium exchange of cells.

Riboflavin is needed for proper adaptability of the eye to light.

Riboflavin helps break down and assimilate carbohydrates, proteins, fats.

Riboflavin is needed for proper assimilation of iron.

Riboflavin helps proper development of muscles (muscle tone) and it is a growth factor.

Goats' milk does not have enough Riboflavin. Children on goats' milk alone become stunted. Brewers yeast should be added.

B₆ or Pyridoxin

B$_6$ is very sensitive to light, but not so much to heat. It is water soluble and is synthesized by a healthy intestinal flora.

1) B$_6$ influences as a coferment the amino acid metabolism.
2) B$_6$ regulates the proper utilization of unsaturated fats.
3) B$_6$ is needed for anabolism and catabolism of tissues as in skin, liver, heart and lungs. (To keep it well nourished.)
4) B$_6$ is needed for the proper activity of the central nervous system.
5) B$_6$ encourages growth of yeast, plant and animals.

If following symptoms persist check with your physician and discuss possible B$_6$ deficiency with him.

> Acne, juveniles
> Arteriosclerosis
> Ear noises
> Eczema in babies
> Epileptic type convulsions in babies and children
> Fainting easily
> Inflammation of lips
> Leukopenia: diminishing of white corpuscles of the blood
> Meniers' syndrome
> Morning sickness
> Motion sickness
> Neuritis from arsenic poison
> Neuritis from toxic condition
> Radiation, side effects of
> Uterine bleeding without pathological disturbances
> Seborrea: particularly on face, lips, mouth
> Tremor a) old age
>   b) rhythmic shaking of muscles
>   c) toxic
> Vomiting after operations
> Whooping cough.

B$_{12}$

B$_{12}$ is synthesized in the healthy intestinal tract, however only in such small amounts that this tiny amount is utilized by the intestinal tract itself and does not reach the liver or the bloodstream.

Scientists tell us that there was a time, many thousands of years ago, when the human body was able to manufacture enough B$_{12}$ and utilize it. Since this ability got lost we have to take in B$_{12}$ with our foods or as food supplements. Since B$_{12}$ is plentiful in muscle meat, and raw milk vegetarians should make it a point to supplement their diets with B$_{12}$ and folic acid.

B$_{12}$ taken in tablet form can only be utilized when an intrinsic factor is present. This "intrinsic factor" is found in healthy stomach juices. It coats and protects B$_{12}$ until it reaches the small intestines, from there it is delivered to the liver and blood stream. In order to assure proper B$_{12}$ intake, Folic acid should be taken with it or injections should be considered.

If following symptoms persist, check with your physcian and discuss with him possible B$_{12}$ deficiencies:

Anemia
Arm-shoulder pain
Appetite, loss of
Burning pains
Concentration, lack of
Depressed feeling
Eczema
Exhaustion
Feeling of deadness
Loss of mental energy
Needle and pins
Numbness
Pain in facial muscles/facial nerves
Pernicious anemia
Polyneuritis (particularly due to alcohol)
Rosacea
Sore mouth
Stiffness, shooting pains
Tired of school.

Vitamin C

The most popular vitamin is Vitamin C. 5,000 tons are manufactured annually. It is a white crystalline powder which is lemon sour. Vitamin C is found in all natural foods, vegetables, fruits, eggs, milk and meat. Every cell of every living organism (plant or animal) is rich in Vitamin C. Vitamin C in food is easily destroyed by exposure to light, heat, air, metals.

The richest natural source for Vitamin C is the acerola cherry. 1/4 lb. of them have 2,000 mg. C. While the same amount of apples have only 20 mg. at the most.

It is strange that the lowly potato becomes important for Vitamin C. When prepared properly it still maintains a great portion of Vitamin C. Raw potatoes are excellent for Vitamin C supply.

Smokers need extra Vitamin C. Each Cigarette destroys 25 mg. of Vitamin C. Nonsmokers subjected to smoke filled offices need the same amount.

Animals are able to manufacture their own Vitamin C with the exceptions of guinea pigs, apes, prairie dogs and deer. The human species lost the ability to manufacture Vitamin C in themselves. However there are known some "freaks" for whom this rule does not stand. Or are these "freaks" the future generation?

Vitamin C possible deficiency symptoms are:
    Anemia
    Bleeding of membranes in mouth
    Bleeding under skin
    Brittle bones
    Changes in heart health
    Edema
    Fatigue
    Loose teeth
    Loss of concentration
    Wounds which do not heal.
Vitamin C is used for:
    Adrenal gland exhaustion
    Burns
    Colds

Ginginits
Hayfever
Infectious diseases
Metal poison
Pigmentation during pregnancy
Rheumatic fever
Rhesus
Shorten time of labor (childbirth)
Stomatitis.
   Vit. C is an activator of cell activity.
   Vit. C is an energizer.
   Vit. C is needed for healthy tissue.
   Vit. C is active in hormone production.
   Vit. C is needed for healthy blood.
   Vit. C is a detoxifier of:
a) metals
b) toxic micro organism
c) self intoxication
d) toxic matter such as tobacco, DDT, stabilizers, food poison and other foreign matters.

Vitamin E

Vitamin E is a fat soluble vitamin which is not synthesized in the body and has to be taken in from outside sources.

Recently it was found that Vitamin E has a structural resemblance of the green pigmentation of plants, the chlorophyll, and the research is in full swing to find out whether the plants build up Vitamin E from and through chlorophyll or not.

We know of Alpha Tocopherol
Beta Tocopherol
Gamma Tocopherol
Delta Tocopherol

The mixed Tocopherol has all forms of Vitamin E in it and research goes on to find out why the mixed tocopherols can influence the glandular system and its hormone production. Meanwhile mankind is happy with the results of Vitamin E.

Vitamin E is an antioxidant. It keeps oils from becoming rancid.

Vitamin E influences the oxidation process of every cell of our body (without oxygen no life).

Vitamin E enhances the action of Vitamin A and makes it easier for the liver to store Vitamin A.

Vitamin E is pretty stable to heat but is destroyed by freezing processes.

Vitamin E deficiency shortens the lifespan of the red blood corpuscles therefore Vitamin E deficiency can be found by special blood tests.

The female needs more Vitamin E than the male. In case following symptoms persist check with your physician and discuss with him the possible Vitamin E deficiencies.

Arteriosclerosis
Circulation impaired
Colitis
Degenerative changes in liver, membranes,
    muscles, skin, tissue

Disc trouble
Exhaustion
General weakness
Heart health
Intestinal ulcers
Miscarriage
Menopause syndrome
Menstrual trouble
Muscle weakness
Stomach ulcers

Vitamin D

Vitamin D is called the sunshine vitamin because the body can manufacture Vitamin D with the ultra violet rays of the sun, when coming in contact with the skin. Deficiency symptoms are known as:

       Lack of vigor inter-changes with restlessness
       Back of head (in babies) perspires while sleeping
       Enlarged joints
       Faulty jaw development
       Bowleggedness
       Retarded growth
       Convulsions

Sources of Vitamin D are:

       Sunshine
       Sunlamps
       Sunflower seeds
       Egg yolk
       Cod liver oil.

Vitamin K

There are 7 different kinds of Vit. K.

K_1 is found in nature: potatoes, spinach, alfalfa, oils and liver.

K_2 is formed by the friendly bacteria in the intestinal tract (importance of healthy flora).

K_3, K_4, K_5, K_6, K_7 are made in chemical laboratories and belong in the hands of experienced physicians and not in nutrition centers.

Vit. K deficiency can occur under following circumstances:

Lack of synthesis in colon

Disfunction of liver

not enough gall, Antibiotica and Sulfonamides

Deficiency symptoms are known as:

Bleeding of subcutanous tissue

Bleeding into muscles

Bleeding into colon

Bleeding of other inner organs.

Choline

Choline is a food substance which a healthy colon rich in good flora manufactures itself.

Whenever following symptoms persist, check with your physician and discuss with him possible choline deficiencies.

Bloatedness

Sluggish liver

has no desire for meat dishes

Hungry but feels full after a few bites

Kidney is bleeding, but no pathological changes can be found in kidney

Cholesterol is elevated but strict diet has no influence on it.

For reducing, choline has proven very helpful in some cases.

Choline is a methyl donor as Vitamin E is and increases the metabolism in general and liver and kidney in particular.

Niacin or Nicotinic Acid

In 1915 America lost 11,000 people to pellagra, a deficiency disease of niacin and B-complex. It was the most dreaded plague of the south, where the staple food was corn and pork fat.

With the discovery of nicotinic acid as the main factor to heal this plague, huge amounts of yeast was given to the unfortunate pellagra diseased population and pellagra, the black tongue disease, became a disease of the past.

Niacin can be synthesized in a healthy environment of the colon. However it needs the presence of B_1, B_2 and B_6 to do so.

If following symptoms persist check with your physician and discuss with him possible deficiencies of Niacin, Nicotinic acid, Niacinamide:

> Alcoholism
> Antiacidity of stomach
> Butterfly eczema
> Celiac disease
> Concentration, loss of
> Confusion
> Depressed feeling
> Eczema
> Enteritis
> Fatigue
> Fear
> Frostbites
> Inflammation of membranes of mouth
> Inflammation of skin when exposed to sun and
>   resembles roses (Mal de la Rose)
> Nervousness
> Neuralgia
> Urticaria
> Tongue deep red with fissures, will turn black
>   when deficiency is great.

Pantothenic Acid

The healthy digestive tract of the human species is able to bring forth enough pantothenic acid. Even enough in stress situations. However, when the intestinal flora is disturbed through antimicrobic procedure and environment, pantothenic acid cannot be produced and is missing.

The active form of pantothenic acid is the coenzyme "A" which is particularly plentiful in bran substance. Pantothenic acid is needed for the normal functioning of tissue and muscles. It protects all membranes from infections. It is needed for the proper function of the endocrine system. It is particularly needed in:

Stress situations
Infections
Overwork
Worries.

Lack of pantothenic acid expresses itself in:

Disturbance of neuromotor system
Physical weakness
Depression
Digestive problems
Sensitivity to infections.

Pantothenic acid is called an anti-graying vitamin.

PART II

Minerals
in Nutrition

Calcium

Of all the minerals, calcium is the one the body has the most of. It is needed for the bones and cartilage, for proper blood clotting, nerve and muscle functioning, hormone formation and many other chemical wonders.

Calcium balance is the key to mineral balance and it is an important factor in health.

Calcium, phosphorus and magnesium have to be in harmony with each other at all times. With this foundation other minerals can formulate in a similar trinity pattern.

If calcium is too low, your toes and legs cramp at night in a painful way. If phosphorus is too low, calcium crystals deposit in joints and muscles which become painful and stiff particularly with weather changes.

In case our body got hold of some heavy metals such as lead, arsenic, even DDT, formaldehyde or mercury, the calcium household becomes heavily disturbed. Other factors come into the proper calcium assimilation and digestion for example, lack of stomach juices and so on.

If the following symptoms persist, check with your physician and discuss with him possible calcium deficiency.

Brooding
Lack of willpower
Lack of courage
Listlessness
Leg cramps at night
Pus formation
Sighing
Soft bones
Sores do not heal
Sour odor
Sleeplessness
Toes cramp at night
Too much salivation

Ugly scars
Complaining about little
   things
Cyst formation
Deformities due to soft
   bones
Difficulty in thinking
Headache, more in
   afternoons
Heart palpitation,
   particularly at night
Heart cramps at night.

Calcium lactate works mainly on muscles; Calcium gluconate on nerves and blood; and Bonemeal calcium on bones.

Fluoride (Calcium)

Calcium fluoride is a constituent of the elastic fibers of the skin, the muscle tissue, the blood vessels, the surface of bones and the teeth. It is something that gives hardness and stability.

In case following symptoms persist, discuss with your physician possible calcium fluoride deficiencies.

> Backwardness in manners
> Brown spots on skin
> Chapped hands
> Eyeball aches
> Eyelids stick in morning
> Dilated blood vessels on legs (varicose veins)
> Arms or inside your body dirty, oily, yellowish skin pigmentation
> Hard crusts form in nose
> Great aversion to darkness
> Puffed, swollen body parts which come and go. It can be on eyes, lips, ankles, abdomen or neck
> Liver trouble
> Spleen enlarged, there are not enough strong fibers to hold it.

All members of the cabbage family are rich in calcium fluoride as:

> Cauliflower
> Sauerkraut
> Chinese cabbage
> Red and green cabbage.

The non-toxic calcium fluoride should not be mistaken for sodium fluoride.

Sodium fluoride is added to city water and is one of the most toxic medicines known to man, only surpassed by Cyanide of Mercury.

Since this booklet deals only with food supplements not with medicine, it is not my job to point out the toxic cumulative effect of above-mentioned medicine.

Iodine

The Medical Dictionary (Dorland) gives following description of Iodine. "A nonmetallic element, a halogen element which is essential in nutrition, being especially abundant in the colloid of the thyroid gland." The higher the altitude the more iodine the body requires. Mount Everest could not be conquered until men took kelp (seaweed) tablets along. American Indians in the high mountains of the Rockies carried kelp as their most prized possession, and they made the long journey to the ocean to trade for kelp and bring it home.

Kelp is iodine with trace minerals. If following symptoms persist, consult with your physician and discuss with him possible iodine deficiencies:
Always cold feeling
Appearance, dull, listless
Dislike for moisture
Dull pains under both shoulder blades
Enlarged glands
Goiter
Headaches, dull
Heart and chest pressure
Little interest in life
Mind slow and dull
Movements slow
Puffy face and body
Pulse alternates often
Swelling of fingers
Swelling of toes.

Iron

Without iron the blood could not hold the valuable oxygen and could not deliver oxygen throughout the body.

If following symptoms persist consult with your physician and discuss with him possible iron deficiencies.

Anemia
Easily fatigued
Crying involuntarily
Dizziness
Difficulty in breathing
Dull hearing
Fault finding tendency
Flattened fingernails
Fissured tongue
Mentally hard to please
Painful breathing
Pains in head (stinging)
Pains in heels
Pains in sole of feet
Pains in fingertips
Pains in shoulder joints
Poor equilibrium
Sleepless at night
Sleepy in daytime

Magnesium

We have about 1 ounce of magnesium in our body. We need it for bones, blood and body fluids.

Magnesium is needed to utilize carbohydrates properly, to make our own protein from amino acids, to maintain our muscles and to keep our hormones going.

If following symptoms persist, check with your physician and discuss with him possible magnesium deficiency.

      Aching neck and shoulder muscles
      Allergy to wool
      Burning sensation in mouth
      Bed wetting
      Chilly after retiring
      Fear
      Grief, apprehension
      Gas and wind in intestine
      Inflated intestine
      Nervous heart palpitation
      Muscle jerk spasms
      Restless movements of eyes and fingers
      Yellowish whites of eyes
      Sensitivity to noise
      Sleep with eyes half open
      Teeth sensitive to cold water
      Tooth ache when nothing is wrong
      Tremors
      Twitching of body
      Winding motion of body.

There are different kinds of magnesium combinations on the market.

Magnesium gluconate is utilized particularly well by nerves. Nerve involvement as fear, nerve twitching, muscle twitching, bet wetting, restlessness, grief, apprehension and so on.

Magnesium phosphate is indicated by cramp-like contraction of muscles.

Magnesium oxide when muscles ache and twist and become stiff. It is a counter player to calcium.

Manganese

Manganese is a yin mineral. It is more needed by the female species of all creatures. The most outstanding symptom is, when the female will reject the offspring. It can be seen at times in cats, dogs and humans as well. Physical signs of manganese deficiencies:

Tenderness in nipples
Glands swell easily
Enlargement of ovaries
Womb falling and protruding
Fainting spells
Mental disagreement to every statement
Crying spells
Dislikes children
Wants to be left alone
Bones crackle when walking (noisy)
Burning sensation in limbs and body
Gripping sensation in limbs and body
Eyes red and swollen.

Phosphorus

Phosphorus is the counterbalance of calcium. It is closely associated with calcium and Vitamin D in the body. It makes up about 1% of the body weight, most of it is in the skeleton. The rest is involved in practically every complex activity of protein, fats and carbohydrates. Phosphorus helps to produce energy, builds new tissue and maintains good structure.

To get enough phosphorus you can rely on meat, fish, vegetables, whole grains, eggs, nuts and legumes.

In case following symptoms persist, check with your physician and discuss with him possible phosphorus deficiencies.

Afraid of tomorrow
Dislike opposite sex
Dislike work
Fearful of the unknown
General weakness
Loss of muscle tone in arms and legs
Numbness in limbs
Paralysis
Prone to bronchitis
Prone to arthritis
Repeated jaundiced condition.

Potassium

Potassium is needed for keeping the chemical balance of the fluids in our cells. In a healthy body, potassium is mainly found inside the cells while sodium rich fluids bathe the cells from the outside. The electrical exchange between potassium and sodium (one having positively charged ions, the other negatively charged ions) brings the nutrients into the cells and takes the waste products from the cells.

If following symptoms persist consult with your physician and discuss with him possible potassium shortage.

Angry-looking sores
Bitter taste in mouth
Constriction of urethra without pathological
   cause
Distention of stomach
Distress of stomach
Distress in pit of stomach
Dropsy
Dry throat
Eczema on feet and legs
Headache in lower back of head
Inability to digest sugar
Itchy dry skin
Kidney function impaired
Liver function impaired
Low grade infection
Muscle weakness
Pyorrhea
Swollen ankles
Swollen ovaries
Swollen testicles
Tendency to blisters
Water retention
Weakness in female organs
Weak ligaments.

Potassium is needed for proper muscle functioning.
Potassium is needed for iron balance.
Potassium is needed for cell nutrition.

Silicon

Silicon is found in all grasses, particularly oatstraw, oats, white onion, radish, calmyrna figs and grains.

Silicon gives strength to bones, nerves, tissue, mucous membrane, hair and nails.

Silicon deficiencies are known to be:
Itchy ears
Sties on eyelids
Ear discharge in children
Ulceration of gums
Ulceration of tongue
Parched lips and fingertips
Toothache without cavities
Teeth sensitive to cold
Tendency to boils
Drug addiction.
Silicon gives mental strength.
Listless
Lack of determination
No ambition to brain work
Nervous exhaustion.

If above symptoms persist, check with your physician and discuss with him possible silicon deficiencies.

Sodium

Sodium is very essential for animals and men alike. Animals are known to trot many miles for "salt licks" and farmers place a "salt lick" in barren or pasture for their animals.

Sodium is in the fluids of the body. It is found outside the body cells. Every cell is bathed in a sodium containing fluid. Here in America it is not often that someone suffers from lack of sodium because table salt is readily available. However, in summer heat, lots of vomiting, excess perspiration, inability of sodium utilization as well as adrenal gland exhaustion. Sodium deficiencies may occur.

In case following symptoms persist, consult with your physician and discuss with him possible sodium deficiencies.

Adrenal gland exhaustion
Bloating
Breath has bad, foul odor
Chlorosis
Collapse with burning face
Confusion of mind
Constipation
Excessive thirst
Exhaustion
Gas in stomach
Getting real angry over little things
Glasses have to be changed too often
Hair is falling out
Hayfever
Hysterical behavior
Indigestion
Loses temper over nothing
Loss of smell
Mental depression
Protein as eggs, meat or fish make gas.

Sulfur

Sulfur is essential in ridding the body of poisonous substances. It is needed for the health of bones, hair, nails and the fluids in our joints and vertebrae discs. We do not need much sulfur but we feel it when we do not have enough.

If following symptoms persist, consult with your physician and discuss with him possible sulfur deficiencies.

Desire to massage and knead the muscles of
arms and legs
Disc trouble
Difficulty in speaking
Difficulty in singing
Fingernails thin
Fingernails split
Hair dull
Joint troubles
Joyless appearance
Prolonged time for regaining strength after
illness or overwork
Pus formation with delayed healing
Menstruation delayed
Menstruation irregular
Moodiness
Sores do not heal
Toxic conditions
Throat is whiter than other parts of neck
Voicebox gives out easily
Women ailments which repeat often.

Zinc

Zinc is needed in wound healing, trauma after surgery, for a healthy pancreas (assists insulin production) and prostate, for a healthy thyroid, thymus and the immune system.

In case the following symptoms persist, check with your physician and discuss with him possible zinc deficiencies.

Eye trouble
Cataract
Earache
Brain trouble
Delirium
Apoplexy
Mania
Epilepsy
Blisters on face and scalp
Gout
Neuralgia.

The missing link for proper zinc utilization is an enzyme hormone called picolinate. Zinc picolinate is a breakthrough in nutrition.

PART III

LOCATOR

Body parts, Symptoms	**Nutrients and Foods**

A

Aches:	
in neck (see Stomach)	
in neck muscle	Magnesium
in shoulder muscle	
Acid indigestion	B_1, B_2, and minerals from raw potatoes
Acid stomach	Niacin, B-Complex
Acidosis	B_1, minerals from raw potatoes
Acne:	
juvenilis (young people)	A, C, B_6
vulgaris (common)	A, C, B_2, E
Adrenal gland	C, B-Complex, Pantothenic acid, Sodium
Afraid of tomorrow	Phosphorus
Alcoholism	B-Complex, B_1, B_{12}, Choline, Inositol, Pantothenic acid, E, Niacin
Allergic to wool	Magnesium
Allergies	A, G, B_6, B_{12}, E, Pantothenic acid, L-Histidine
Always cold	Iodine
Anemia	A, B_2, B_6, B_{12}, Copper, Iron, Manukka raisins and molasses for extra minerals
Anus: itching (see Liver)	
Appearance dull	Iodine
Arm-shoulder syndrome (pain)	B-Complex, B_{12}, Folic acid
Arteriosclerosis (hardening of arteries)	A, B_{12}, E, Lecithin, distilled water
Arthritis	A, B-Complex, B_1,& B_{15}, D, E, Trace minerals from alfalfa seeds (trace)

Body parts, Symptoms	Nutrients and Foods
Arthritis (continued)	(Check alkalinity. When too acid, add phosphorus and magnesium to your diet. When too alkaline, add calcium, protein from pumpkin seeds to your diet and take okra tablets for extra minerals.)
Asthma	A, C, B-Complex, Choline & Inositol, Lecithin, E
Athlete's foot	A, follow suggestion on your Clorox bottle
Aversion to darkness	Calcium fluoride

B

Backwardness in manners	Calcium fluoride
Balding	Paba, Biotin, Folic acid, Inositol
Bedsores	C, E, Copper
Bedwetting	B_1, B-Complex, E, Magnesium
Bitter taste in mouth	Potassium
Bladder	A, B_6, Magnesium
Bladder infection	A, B_6, C, E, Trace minerals from Uva Ursi
Bleeding gums	C, E, P, K_2
Blister on eye	B_1
Bloatedness	Choline, Sodium
Blood pressure low	B_1, B_6, B-Complex, Copper, Iron, Niacin
Blood pressure high	Lecithin, B_1, B-Complex, Garlic for the elasticity of the vessels
Blurred vision	B_6
Boils	A, C, Bioflavonoids, E
Bones brittle	B-Complex, Bone meal for calcium, B_{12}, C, E

Body parts, Symptoms	Nutrients and Foods
Bones, crackle when walking	Manganese
Breath has bad, foul odor	Sodium
Brooding	Calcium
Brown spots on skin	Calcium fluoride
Bruises	C, Bioflavonoids, Panto-thenic acid, K_2 from chestnut leaves or alfalfa
Burning feet	B_6, B-Complex, Panto-thenic acid, E, Copper, Iron
Burning pains	B_{12}
Burning sensation in body and limbs	Manganese, B_{12}
Burns	C, E
Butterfly eczema	Niacin, B-Complex, Soy oil

C

Callus	A, C
Canker sores	B_6, Niacin, B_2
Carbuncles	A, B-Complex, C, E
Cataract	A, B_2, B-Complex, C, E, trace minerals from Angelica root
Celiac disease	B from rice polishings, Folic acid, Calcium, Magnesium, Niacin
Chapped hands	Calcium fluoride, Silicon
Chilly after retiring	Magnesium
Chlorosis	Sodium
Cholesterol	C, Bioflavonoids, B-Complex, E, F, Choline, Inositol, Magnesium, Lecithin
Chorea	A, B_1, B_6, Magnesium

Body parts, Symptoms	Nutrients and Foods
Cirrhosis of liver	A, B-Complex, Choline, Inositol, B_{12}, C, E, Magnesium
Clots	C, E, Bioflavonoids, Rutin & minerals from white oak bark tea
Collapse, with burning face	Sodium
Colds	A, C, Iodine, Calcium, Trace minerals from elderflower and peppermint
Colitis	A, C, B-Complex from rice polishings, E, F, Magnesium, Potassium from bran, Trace minerals from white oak bark and goldenseal root.
Colon, peristaltic movement impaired	Pantothenic acid
Complaining about little things	Calcium
Concentration, loss of	B_{12}, B-Complex, Glutamic acid, Niacin
Confusion	Niacin, C, B-Complex
Confusion of mind	Sodium
Conjunctivitis	B_2
Constipation	B, C, Sodium, Trace minerals
Constriction of urethra	Potassium
Corns	A
Cramps in legs	Calcium lactate, B_1
Cramps, menstrual	Calcium lactate, B_1
Crying, involuntary	Calcium
Crying spells	Manganese
Cyst formation	Calcium
Cystitis (see Bladder inflammation)	

Body parts, Symptoms	Nutrients and Foods

D

Dandruff	F
Deafness	A, B_{12}, E, F, Iodine, Niacin
Deformities due to soft bones	Calcium
Delirium tremens	B_1
Depressed feeling	Niacin, B-Complex, B_{12}, C, E
Dermatitis	B_2, B_6, B-Complex, E, F
Desire to stretch frequently	Calcium
Diabetes	B_1, B_2, B_6, B_{12}, Niacin, C, E, Lecithin, Potassium
Diarrhea, chronic	B_6, C, F, Calcium, Magnesium
Difficulty in speaking and singing	Sulfur
Difficulty in taking a deep breath	Iron
Difficulty in thinking	Calcium
Dilated blood vessel on legs (veins)	Calcium fluoride
Dirty, oily yellowish skin pigmentation	Calcium fluoride
Disc trouble	E, B-Complex, C, Pantothenic acid, B_{12}, Sulfur
Dislike of children	Manganese
Dislike of opposite sex	Phosphorus
Dislike of moisture	Iodine
Dislike of work	Phosphorus
Distention of stomach	Potassium
Distraction by noise	B-Complex from rice bran, E, Folic acid, F, Iron, Sulfur, Magnesium
Diverticulitis	B-Complex from rice bran, E, Folic acid, F, Iron, Sulfur, Magnesium

Body parts, Symptoms	Nutrients and Foods
Dizziness	B₁, B₁₂, C, Niacin, Calcium, Iron
Dry skin	A, C, E, F
Dry throat	Potassium
Dropsy	Potassium, C, E
Dull pains under both shoulder blades	Iodine

E

Ear noises	A, B-Complex, B₆, C and P
Easily fatigued	Iron
Eczema	A, B-Complex, B₆, B₁₂, C, D, F, Calcium, Magnesium, Niacin
Eczema, baby	B₆
Eczema, feet and legs	Potassium
Edema	B₆, C, Potassium
Emphysema	A, B-Complex, C, E, Folic acid, Friendly bacteria, Aloe Vera juice for trace minerals
Enlarged glands	Iodine, C, B-Complex, F, Pantothenic acid, Lettuce water for trace minerals
Enlarged joints	D, Calcium
Enlarged liver, spleen, uterus (without pathological changes)	Calcium fluoride
Enlarged ovaries	E, Manganese
Enteritis	B-Complex from rice bran, B₂, Friendly bacteria, Oak bark tea for trace minerals, niacin
Epileptic type of convulsive disorder	B₆, Calcium, Magnesium

Body parts, Symptoms	Nutrients and Foods
Exhaustion	B-Complex, B_{12}, C, E, F, Pantothenic acid
Eyeballs ache	Calcium fluoride
Eyes burning	A, B_2, Eyebright herb for trace minerals
Eye fibrillation	B_1
Eye lids:	
chronic infection	A, B-Complex, C, Calcium
glued in the morning	A
stick in the morning	Calcium fluoride
spasm	B_2
Eyes, red and swollen	Manganese
Eye strain	A, B_2, C, E
Eyes, tired	A, B_2, C, E, Eyebright for trace minerals
Excessive thirst	Sodium
Exhaustion	Sodium, C, B-Complex, Pantothenic acid

F

Fainting spell	E, B-Complex, B_6, Manganese
Fatigue, chronic	A, B-Complex, B_{12}, C, E, Pantothenic acid, Niacin, Folic acid , Trace minerals
Fatty liver	A, B-Complex, B_{12}, C, E, Choline, Inositol, Lecithin, Sulfur as sulfur baths, Trace minerals from buckthorn tea
Fault finding tendency	Iron
Fear	Niacin, B-Complex, C, Magnesium
Fear of the unknown	Phosphorus
Feet, burning	B-Complex, C, E, Pantothenic acid, Copper
Feet, feeling of deadness	B_{12}

Body parts, Symptoms	Nutrients and Foods
Fever	A, C, Bioflavonoids, Calcium lactate, Trace minerals from juice of raw potatoes
Fever blisters	B_2
Fingernails, flattened	Iron
Fingernails, thin	Sulfur
Fingernails, split	Sulfur
Fissured tongue	Iron, B-Complex
Fissures in corner of mouth	B_2
Frostbite	K_2 from alfalfa, Niacin

G

Gas, in stomach and intestines	Sodium, Magnesium
Gastritis (inflammation of stomach lining)	A, B-Complex from rice polishings, E, F, Lecithin, Trace minerals from flax seed tea
Getting really angry over little things	Sodium
Gingivitis	C, Bioflavonoids
Glands (see Enlarged glands)	
Glaucoma	A, B-complex, B_2, C, Bioflavonoids, E. (Restrict sweets as your physician tells you to.)
Globulin deficiency	Pantothenic acid
Goiter	A, B-Complex, Calcium, Kelp
Gout	B-Complex, C, E, Pantothenic Acid, Sour cherries for minerals
Grief, apprehension	Magnesium
Gripping sensation in limbs	Manganese

Body parts, Symptoms	Nutrients and Foods
	H
Hair	A, B-Complex, F, Kelp for trace minerals
Hair, brittle	A
Hair, dull	Sulfur
Hair, graying	C, E, B-Complex, Folic acid, B_{12}, Paba, Pantothenic acid, Copper, Kelp
Hair, oily	B_2
Hair, falling	Sodium
Halitosis (bad breath)	B-Complex, Choline, Inositol, Chlorophyll
Hard crusts form in nose	Calcium fluoride
Hay fever	A, B-Complex, C, Pantothenic acid, Sodium
Headaches, dull	Iodine
Headaches in lower back of head	Potassium
Headaches, more in the afternoons	Calcium
Hearing, dull	Iron
Heart	E, B-Complex, C, Magnesium, Calcium, Lecithin
Heart, cramps at night	Calcium
Heart, enlarged	B_1
Heart, extra beats	B_1
Heart, too fast	B_1
Heart, palpitation at night	Calcium
Heart and chest pressure	Iodine
Hemorrhoids	B_6, Calcium, Chlorophyll
Herpes Zester	B-Complex, Chlorophyll, B-Complex, B_1, Magnesium, Calcium
Hungry, but feeling full after a few bites	Choline

Body parts, Symptoms	Nutrients and Foods
Hyper insulinism	A, B-Complex, C, Pantothenic acid, Zinc, Sulfur from hops tea
Hysterical behavior	Sodium

I

Impetigo (pimples filled with pus)	A, E, Folic acid
Inability to digest sugar	B_2, Potassium
Indigestion	Sodium
Infection, low grade	Sulfur
Infection, tendency to	A, C, D, E, Bioflavonoids, Calcium lactate, Minerals from fresh lemon juice
Inflammation of lips	B_6
Inflammation of mouth	Niacin
Inflammation of muscles	C, E, Pantothenic acid
Inflated intestines	Magnesium
Influenza	A, C, B-Complex, Pantothenic acid, Minerals from linden blossom tea and mint tea
Insomnia (sleeplessness)	B_6, D, Calcium lactate, Minerals from catnip or valerian root.
Itchy dry skin	Potassium

J

Joint trouble	Sulfur
Joyless appearance	Sulfur

K

Kidney	A, B-Complex, C, Magnesium, Trace minerals from herb teas such as watermelon seed tea, Couchgrass, Cornsilk, Uva Ursi

Body parts, Symptoms	Nutrients and Foods
Kidney, bleeding	(see Choline)
Kidney, function impaired	Potassium
Kidney stones	A, B-Complex, Stone root tea for minerals

L

Labor pain	B_1, Calcium lactate
Labor, prolonged	B_1
Labyrinthitis (inner ear)	C, Bioflavonoids, B-Complex, B_{12}, Folic acid, E
Leg cramps at night	Calcium
Leukopenia (diminishing of white blood corpuscles)	B_6
Listlessness	Calcium
Little interest in life	Iodine
Liver problems	A, C, E, Potassium, Choline, Inositol
Loose teeth	C, Bioflavonoids
Lose temper over nothing	Sodium
Loss of alkali reserves	B_1
Loss of appetite	B_6, B_{12}
Loss of appetite for meat dishes	Choline
Loss of breath, under slightest exercise	B_1
concentration	B_{12}, Folic acid
courage	C, Calcium
energy	B-Complex, B_1, Lecithin, Pantothenic acid
eyesight from tobacco	B_{12}, Folic acid
eyesight from diabetes	Zinc, Paprika
hearing	A
ligament reflexes	B-Complex, B, E
mental energies	B_{12}
muscle tone	Phosphorus

Body parts, Symptoms	Nutrients and Foods
Loss of (continued)	
sense of smell	A, Sodium
stomach acidity	B_1, B-Complex, Niacin
strength in muscles of arms and legs	B_1
taste	A
tear secretion	B-Complex, Kelp for trace minerals
willpower	Calcium
Low grade infection	Potassium
Lumbago	B-Complex, B_1

M

Measles	C, Warmth, Minerals from raw potatoes (grated)
Men developing female breasts	B_1. (Estrogen gets upset with lack of B_1.)
Meniers syndrome	B-Complex, B_6, B_1, B_{12}, C, E, F, Niacin, Potassium, Bioflavonoids
Menopause	(Try Vitamin E which is food for the master gland, the pituitary. If this does nothing for you try B-Complex from rice bran, Calcium, Vitamin D, **Red Bone Marrow.**)
Menstrual flow, excessive	B-Complex, B_{12}, E, Folic acid, Iron, Trace minerals from okra
Menstrual flow, irregular	B-Complex, E, Folic acid, Sulfur, Trace minerals from fireweed
Mental depression	Sodium
Mentally hard to please	Iron
Metal poison	C, Okra, Squash

Body parts, Symptoms	Nutrients and Foods
Mind dull and slow	Iodine
Mononucleosis	B-Complex, B_6, C, E, Pantothenic acid, Copper, Trace minerals from lettuce water and raspberry leaf tea
Morning sickness	B_6, Trace minerals from peach leaves
Moodiness	Sulfur
Motion sickness	B_6
Muscle cramps	B_1, B_2, E, Calcium lactate
Muscle function	E
Muscle pain	B, E, Calcium lactate
Muscle weakness	Potassium
Muscle jerk	Magnesium
Muscle spasms (if spasms are in daytime)	Magnesium
Muscle spasms (if spasms are at night)	Calcium lactate
Muscular dystrophy	A, B_6, B_{12}, E, C, B-Complex, Choline, Inositol, Pantothenic acid
Multiple sclerosis	B-Complex, E, C, B, B_{15}, Lecithin, Niacin, Magnesium, Pantothenic acid

N

Body parts, Symptoms	Nutrients and Foods
Nails	A, Calcium
Nails which do not grow	B_2
Nearsightedness	A, B-Complex, C, E
Needles and pins	B_{12}, Folic acid
Nephritis	A, B_2, B_6, Choline, Inositol, Lecithin, Calcium, Magnesium, Potassium, Trace minerals from herb teas

Body parts, Symptoms	Nutrients and Foods
Nervous heart palpitation	B-Complex, B_6, Lecithin, Magnesium, Calcium, Trace minerals from Valerian root
Nervousness	Magnesium, Lecithin, Calcium, B-Complex, B_6
Neuritis, caused by arsenic poison	B_6, Niacin
Neuritis, caused by alcohol, lead, drug poison	B-Complex, B_6, Niacin, Trace minerals from okra, Pumpkin
Neuritis of eye	B-Complex, B_1
Neuritis in lower extremities	B_6, Niacin, B-Complex
Neuritis without known cause	B-Complex, B_1, B_{15}, B_6, B_{12}, Lecithin, Pantothenic acid, C-Complex
Night blindness	A
Nose bleed	C, Bioflavonoids, B_{15}, B-Complex, Iron, K_2 from alfalfa, Trace minerals from okra

O

Osteo arthritis	B-Complex, B_1, B_{12}, B_{15}, C, E, Bioflavonoids, Bonemeal for calcium
Osteoporosis	B-Complex, B_{12}, C, D, Calcium, Magnesium, Phosphorus, Bonemeal and kelp for trace minerals
Ovary weak	B-Complex, C-Complex, Copper, Iron, Silicon

Body parts, Symptoms	Nutrients and Foods
Overweight	B-Complex, B_2, B_6, E, C, Iron, Trace minerals from kelp, Choline, Inositol, Potassium from apple vinegar
Overwork	B-Complex, C, Pantothenic acid

P

Pain,	
burning	B_{12}, Folic acid
facial muscle	B_{12}, Folic acid
shoulder–arm syndrome	Iron, Copper, B_{12}, Folic acid
stump (amputated leg)	B_1, B_{12}
Painful breathing	Iron
Painful piles	Silicon
Pains in fingertips	Iron
Pains in head	Iron
Pains in heels	Iron, Copper
Paralysis, curacale (muscle)	Pantothenic acid
Paralysis of facial muscles	B_{12}, Folic acid
Phlebitis	C, E, Bioflavonoids, Trace minerals from white oak bark tea
Photophobia	A, B_2
Pigmentation of skin	A, C, E
Pyorrhea	A, B-Complex, B_6, C, Bioflavonoids, Niacin, Calcium, Potassium
Polyneuritis of toxic nature	B-Complex, B_6, B_{12}, C
Polyps	A, Silicon
Poor equilibrium	Iron, B-Complex, C
Premenstrual tension	A
Prevention against mosquito bites	B_1, B_6
Prostate gland enlarged	A, B-Complex, C, E, F, Potassium, Trace minerals from fenugreek tea

Body parts, Symptoms	Nutrients and Foods
Protein as fish, meat and eggs make gas	Sodium
Prone to arthritis	Phosphorus
Prone to bronchitis	Phosphorus
Puffy face	Iodine
Puffy, swollen parts of the body which come and go	Calcium fluoride
Pulse alternates often	Iodine
Pus formation	A, C, Calcium, Sulfur

R

Radiation, side effects of	B_6
Restlessness	B-Complex, B_1, B_6, Calcium lactate
Restless movements of eyes	Magnesium
Restless movements of fingers	Magnesium
Repeated jaundiced condition	Phosphorus
Retina bleeding	C, Bioflavonoids, Rutin, B_1
Rheumatism	B-Complex, B, B_{15}, C, Bioflavonoids, Folic acid, Calcium in many cases but not all
RH factor	B-Complex, C, Bio-flavonoids, Enzymes from raw foods
Rickets	D, C, Calcium, Kelp baths
Rosacea	B_{12} (Red nose)

S

Sciatica	B-Complex, B_1, B_{15}
Scurvy	C, Bioflavonoids
Seborrhea on face, lips, mouth	B_6

Body parts, Symptoms	Nutrients and Foods
Seborrheic dermatitis	A, B-Complex, Biotin
Sensitive to noise	Magnesium
Shingles	B-Complex, B_1, B_{12}, Folic acid
Sighing	Calcium
Sinus	A, C, Bioflavonoids
Skin red and scaly	A, B_2
Sleeplessness	B, Calcium, Magnesium
Sleeplessness at night, sleepy in daytime	Iron
Sleep with eyes half open	Magnesium
Soft bones	Calcium
Soles of feet itch	Silicon
Sore mouth	B-Complex, B_{12}, Phosphorus
Sore thighs	Silicon
Sores do not heal	Calcium, Sulfur, C, B-Complex
Sour odor	Calcium
Sprue	A, B-Complex from rice polishings, Folic acid, Lecithin
Sterility	A, B-Complex, E
Stiffness with shooting pains	B_{12}
Stomach ulcers	A from carrots–carotene; B from rice polishings, E, C, Bioflavonoids, K_2, Aloe Vera juice for trace minerals
Strengthen colon	B_1
Strengthen memory	A, B-Complex, C, E, Pantothenic acid, Silicon, Glutamic acid
Strengthen muscle	E, Silicon
Stress	A, B-Complex, B_{12}, Folic acid, C, E, Calcium, D,

Body parts, Symptoms	Nutrients and Foods
Stress (continued)	Phosphorus, Pantothenic acid
Stretch marks	E ointment
Stroke	C, Bioflavonoids, E, Choline, Potassium
Sunburn	A, Calcium without D, Paba ointment
Swollen ankles	Potassium
Swollen ovaries	Potassium, fireweed for trace minerals
Swollen testicles	Potassium, trace minerals from fenugreek seeds
Swollen toes and fingers	Iodine

T

Tears:	
excessive	B_2
not enough	B_1
Teeth: sensitive to cold	Magnesium
Throat:	
dry	B_2
too much saliva	Calcium
appears whiter under the chin than on other parts of the neck	Manganese, Sulfur
Thrombosis	C_1, Bioflavonoids, Rutin, E, Trace minerals from white oak bark tea
Tired of school	B_{12}
Toes cramp at night	Calcium
Tongue:	
deep red with fissures	Niacin, B-Complex
painful	B_2
purple red	B_2
Toothache when nothing is wrong	Magnesium
Toxicity	Sulfur

Body parts, Symptoms	Nutrients and Foods
Tremors	Magnesium

U

Ugly scars	Calcium, E
Ulcers	B-Complex, B_{12}, Folic acid, C, E, Iron, K_2 from alfalfa
Underactive thyroid	A, B-Complex, C, E, Choline, Iodine, Trace minerals from kelp
Urticaria	Niacin
Uterine bleeding	B_6 when no other pathological disturbance can be found

V

Vaginal discharge	A, B-Complex, B_2, B_6, C, E, Iron, Trace minerals
Varicose veins	B-Complex, C, Bioflavonoids, E, Trace minerals from white oak bark, Silicon
Voice box gives out	Sulfur
Virus infection	C, Bioflavonoids, A, Trace minerals from sweet basil and lettuce water
Vitality low	B-Complex, B_1, C, E, Pantothenic acid

W

Warts	A, E, Silicon
Water retention	Potassium
Weak ligaments	Potassium, E, C
Weakness in female	Potassium
Whopping cough	B_6
Winding motion of body	Magnesium
Without joy	Sulfur
Women's ailments (repeatedly)	Sulfur

References

American Illustrated Medical Dictionary, Dorland

Feel Like A Million, K. Elwood

Let's Eat Right To Keep Fit, A. Davis

Let's Live, magazine issues 1962–1972

Natureilkunde, Prof. Brauchle

Naturheil praxis, monthly magazine (German), issues 1962–1972

Vitamine bauen uns auf, Heinz Scholz

Vitamins in Medicine, B. & Prescott (England)

Webster dictionary

and scientists and Boulder and professors from the University of Colorado who graciously answered my many questions about how and why minerals and vitamins work.

Books by Hanna

"Wholistic health represents an attitude toward well being which recognizes that we are not just a collection of mechanical parts, but an integrated system which is physical, mental, social and spiritual."

Ageless Remedies from Mother's Kitchen

You will laugh and be amazed at all that you can do in your own pharmacy, the kitchen. These time tested treasures are in an easy to read, cross referenced guide. (94 pages)

Allergy Baking Recipes

Easy and tasty recipes for cookies, cakes, muffins, pancakes, breads and pie crusts. Includes wheat free recipes, egg and milk free recipes (and combinations thereof) and egg and milk substitutes. (34 pages)

Alzheimer's Science and God

This little booklet provides a closer look at this disease and presents Hanna's unique religious perspectives on Alzheimer's disease. (15 pages)

Arteriosclerosis and Herbal Chelation

A booklet containing information on Arteriosclerosis causes, symptoms and herbal remedies. An introduction to the product *Circu Flow.* (17 pages)

Cancer: Traditional and New Concepts

A fascinating and extremely valuable collection of theories, tests, herbal formulas and special information pertaining to many facets of this dreaded disease. (65 pages)

Cookbook for Electro-Chemical Energies

The opening of this book describes basic principles of healthy eating along with some fascinating facts you may not have heard before. The rest of this book is loaded with delicious, healthy recipes. A great value. (106 pages)

God Helps Those That Help Themselves

This work is a beautifully comprehensive description of the seven basic physical causes of disease. It is wholistic information as we need it now. A truly valuable volume. (263 pages)

Good Health Through Special Diets

This book shows detailed outlines of different diets for different needs. Dr. Reidlin, M.D. said, "The road to health goes through the kitchen not through the drug store," and that's what this book is all about. (121 pages)

Hanna's Workshop

A workbook that brings together all of the tools for applying Hanna's testing methods. Designed with 60 templates that enable immediate results.

How to Counteract Environmental Poisons

A wonderful collection of notes and information gleaned from many years of Hanna's teachings. This concise and valuable book discusses many toxic materials in our environment and shows you how to protect yourself from them. It also presents Hanna's insights on how to protect yourself, your family and your community from spiritual dangers. (53 pages)

Instant Herbal Locator

This is the herbal book for the do-it-yourself person. This book is an easy cross referenced guide listing complaints and the herbs that do the job. Very helpful to have on hand. (122 pages)

Instant Vitamin-Mineral Locator

A handy, comprehensive guide to the nutritive values of vitamins and minerals. Used to determine bodily deficiencies of these essential elements and combinations thereof, and what to do about these deficiencies. According to your symptoms, locate your vitamin and mineral needs. A very helpful guide. (55 pages)

New Dimensions in Healing Yourself

The consummate collection of Hanna's teachings. An unequated volume that compliments all of her other books as well as her years of teaching. (155 pages)

Old Time Remedies for Modern Ailments

A collection of natural remedies from Eastern and Western cultures. There are 20 fast cleansing methods and many ways to rebuild your health. A health classic. (115 pages)

Parasites: The Enemy Within

A compilation of years of Hanna's studies with parasites. A rare treasure and one of the efforts to expose the truths that face us every day. (65 pages)

The Pendulum, the Bible and Your Survival

A guide booklet for learning to use a pendulum. Explains various aspects of energy, vibrations and forces. (22 pages)

The Seven Spiritual Causes of Ill Health

This book beautifully reveals how our spiritual and emotional states have a profound effect on our physical well being. It addresses fascinating topics such as Karma, Gratitude, Trauma, Laughter as medicine . . . and so much more. A wonderful volume full of timeless treasures. (142 pages)